D0423037

this

is a

story

about

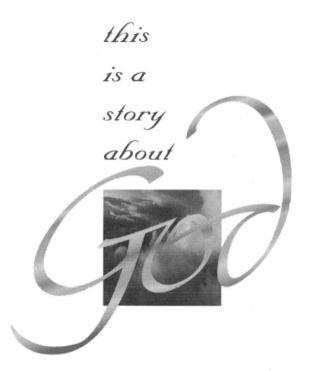

this

is a

story

about

the true account

of two men, an

impossible surgery

and the God of

the universe.

ann kiemel anderson

Beacon Hill Press of Kansas City
Kansas City, Missouri

9312687

Copyright 1998
by Beacon Hill Press of Kansas City

ISBN 083-411-7312

Printed in the
United States of America

Cover Design: Paul Franitza
Photo by: Tony Stone Images/John Turner

Scripture quotations are taken from the *Holy Bible,* New Living Translation,
copyright © 1996. Used by permission of Tyndale House Publishers, Inc.,
Wheaton, Illinois 60189. All rights reserved.

Library of Congress Cataloging-in-Publication Data

Anderson, Ann Kiemel.
   This is a story about God : the true account of two men, an impossible
surgery, and the God of the universe / Ann Kiemel Anderson.
      p.   cm.
   ISBN 0-8341-1731-2 (HB)
     1. Nash, David.   2. Liver—Transplantation—Patients—United
States—Religious life.   3. Christian biography—United States. I. Title.
BR1725.N33N43   1998
277.3'0829'0922—dc21
   [B]   97-47014
                                                CIP

10 9 8 7 6 5 4 3 2

to Jesus who gave

His life for us—

and to serafino who

willingly allowed God

to take his life so another

man could live—

*Got any rivers you think
are uncrossable?
Got any mountains you
can't tunnel through?
God specializes in things
thought impossible.
And He will do what no
other power can do.* *

*Copyright © 1945 by Singspiration Music/ASCAP. All rights reserved. Used by permission.

this

is a

story

about

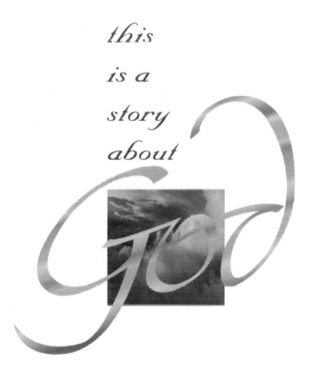

this is a story about God.
the individuals portrayed are real.
the events, current and authentic.
the miracles, all created
    by the only One who can
    author such events.

i am merely an onlooker.
    a first cousin to the main character.
    a friend to the physicians.

this is a story about God.
    about His majestic sweep of love
    and mercy . . . of compassion and
    kindness and extraordinary
    consideration for one man in
    a destitute place.

this is a story about God's touch
    and a sense of pity that so
    enveloped this particular crisis
    that the saga ended with a
    shout of victory. a real-life
    drama covered with fairy-tale wonder.

ultimately, this is a story about

God's infinite power and victory

over evil. there is a darkness

that lurks in and around

people's hearts and lives. a

proclivity to hate, despair,

hopelessness, and the very destruction

of joy and health. a leaning

toward meanness and subtle

deceptions. our natural tendencies

are to be fickle in our approaches

and whimpering in our pursuits.

God's passion for goodness and victory

carries such magnitude that

in time, evil is conquered. evil

may appear to reign in the

affairs of our lives for a time,

but *never* can it conquer us

if God is on our side.

this is a true story, with the same implications for anyone whose own gushing darkness consumes them.

in these pages you will watch

    God melt mountains . . .

    tame dragons of doubt . . . and offer

    cool water for parched,

    thirsty souls that have always

    sought, yet not found, relief

    from life's impossible dilemmas.

always, *this is a story about God*

    and His ultimate power over evil.

    because of God, evil will *never* prevail.

the year: 1958

the place: Carrini, Sicily

the event: the birth of serafino

           healthy, fine baby boy

           youngest of four

in this obscure corner of the world,

    God allowed serafino life. in God's

    scheme of things, a miraculous

    journey was set in motion that only

    the Lord of the universe could understand.

    this boy child would one day offer

life to several who, in different
ways, were losing theirs.

at 10 years of age, serafino's father died
of a brain tumor. through the years,
he was haunted by this loss,
always longing to have known his
father better.

eventually, his mother came to america.
serafino, by then cared for by his aunt,
came across the world to join his
mother. he was 15 years old.

a gentle man. a simple man. an
honorable man. he lived with dignity.
he never spoke ill of others. he
worked hard. he was honest.

in an italian restaurant in chicago,
serafino started making pizza. not
speaking a word of english, he was
constantly attempting to pick up a
few words here and there. a waitress
who worked in the same pizza parlor . . .
miki . . . loved the twinkle in his eyes,
and his easy disposition. she found

herself helping him with simple phrases
and words. though a little older than
serafino, she was attracted to him.
for years, this petite redhead had
prayed for a man who would truly
love her and cherish her. a tall order,
but not too tall for the God of the
universe.

serafino and miki wed. they had a son,
frank. they bought a home and shared
many memories. they were happy.
very in love. contented to embrace
just the simple pleasures and grow
old together. that was their plan.
God had a much nobler, heroic, yet
difficult, destiny for them.

three years before serafino's birth
in Sicily, a pale, but hardy, redheaded
boy baby was born in topeka, kansas. david.
also the youngest of four, his father
was a minister. he rode bikes,
teased his sister and cousins, got

into mischief constantly. a "dennis
the menace" in the family. as he
moved into adolescence, he had
some real growth spurts . . . did
well in basketball and football . . . com-
pleted college and graduate school.
married. had two young children.

in God's Divine order of things,
david became a minister as his
father had been. he loved people.
he visited the sick. stood by
families when their loved ones
died. loved life. now pastoring a
church two hours from chicago, this
6'6" redhead knew that God was great,
life was full, the future bright.
like serafino, however, the Almighty
had assigned a mission to david
and his family. in an incredible
set of circumstances, these two
families' destinies would cross.
would be linked to each other
forever.

this is a story about God. about
    God's redemption for all people.
    everywhere. about His power to
    place people in God-ordained places
    for God-ordained purposes.

like ships passing in the night, we are
    all placed, divinely, like chess pieces on
    a world-sized board. in hospitals,
    neighborhoods, parking lots . . . through
    acquaintances and distant relatives . . .
    in the workplace . . . and sometimes
    even through a stranger on the street, God
    weaves miracles. puts lives together.
    opens doors. changes the world.
    no accidents. no mistakes. no chaos.
    with God, there is *always* order,
    precision, exact timing, and honor.

*God is infinite. He placed the stars
to shine, the tides to come and go,
the heart to love, and the smallest
child to believe in a dream.*

it was no accident that david and
his family had been called from
nashville to pastor a church close
to chicago. and for serafino to be a
couple hours away. there was *no*
connection between the two families. one
protestant, one catholic. one italian,
the other anglo-saxon. these families
did not have one single friend in
common. not any similarities.

yet God, who knows the end from the
beginning, had a plan.

awesome God.
awesome love.
awesome.

it was an ordinary day as most
days are before suddenly, unexpectedly,
one comes face-to-face with news that
alters one's entire destiny.
nashville, tennessee. david was in
graduate school. pastoring a
church. a sharp pain . . . sudden . . . on his
right side.

tests run. serious results.
    cirrhosis of the liver. the worst
    possible diagnosis. deadly.
    the result of medications administered
    to him in his youth for colitis.

the day was no longer ordinary.
    the sun no longer bright.
    the laughter stopped.
    the future joys suddenly
    blasted by one simple diagnosis.

but
    this is a story about God.
    about grace and courage and
    power flowing from God's heart
    into the very fiber of our
    inadequate human longings.

God allows towering obstacles to be
    tossed across our paths so His
    integrity and strength and miraculous
    wonders can shine. can transform
    our quivering doubts into streams
    of shining radiance.

God brings us to the end of all our
human resources so He can
quietly take over and cast out the
mediocrity and deceptiveness in our
thinking. jar it all apart. strip
the crooked foundations of our
hearts. then, in quiet, magnificent
gentleness, He changes us.

*the very day before, we
took for granted. but today we
hold in sacred reverence.*

where we
have grown grumpy . . . complaining . . .
pitying . . . we now recognize our
wretched smallness. the simple gifts
of sunsets and gentle smiles and
a future that takes hold of our hearts.

david was sent to the university of
illinois at chicago (UIC) hospital. dr. layden,
a specialist in liver diseases, was
waiting to see him.

in a small waiting room, with the
smell of popcorn, david waited. who

was this doctor? what did he look
like? a man in a drab brown suit, un-
polished shoes, uncombed hair, and
a bag of popcorn in his hand walked
in. he was unaffected, straightforward.
david had one option: to live one day at
a time and wait. one year, five years.
or never. but only a liver transplant
would save his life.

thus began the saga for david and
his family. a road that would lead one of
two ways. one way, to dream dreams and set
goals for the future. the other way,
to wrap up within a few months a
closure to all that would never be.

forty-five minutes away, in a
chicago suburb, serafino and his
small family were building toward
the future. wanting for frank, their
17-year-old son, a future even better than
theirs.

how do they fit together?
how can God possibly bring good
out of devastation and chaos?
how?

this could be your story. your
>   *question to God. the circumstances*
>   *may be different, but God is not.*
>   *He is changeless and never failing.*
>   *His kaleidoscope of plans and*
>   *answers for you are alive and*
>   *in progress. tell God what you*
>   *need today!*

there lives an uncommon courage in
>   the heart of anyone who must
>   fight to live . . . and an insatiable
>   drive in those who live to help them.

God handpicked a man for a mission,
>   and the team to assist and inspire.
>   He used the exact blend of hearts
>   and minds and human experience to
>   carry out His purposes.

thus it was that david was
>   called. called to work a long,
>   arduous, and often very discouraging
>   mission. and thus it was
>   that the transplant team of the
>   university of illinois at chicago . . . out
>   of all the transplant teams in the
>   world . . . was appointed to assist.

this is no ordinary team of
    doctors. one of the top transplant
    teams in the world, they stood
    in sharp contrast to many physicians
    today. i found a humble
    group of three men and a
    woman who appeared completely
    unlikely to have carved such
    accolades in the medical community.

dr. thomas layden, professor of medicine
    and chief section of digestive and
    liver diseases, was raised irish
    catholic. donning a frayed suit and
    disheveled hair, dr. layden commands
    the final authority for who will
    receive the next liver, and
    when.

dr. wiley is the heart of the team.
    young, gentle-spoken, and black.
    dr. thelma wiley is a born-again
    Christian. her gentle eyes shine with
    unabashed sincerity. the doctor who
    offers comfort, solace, and
    encouragement when patients become
    tentative and fearful. she is the

gentle thread woven through the sea
of fine-tuned technicality and
timing. a smile. a hug. a thoughtful
"you can make it" pep talk
can transform a scared, broken
spirit into one of towering strength
and determination. thus thelma, in
her gracious, unrushed demeanor,
fulfills her part in the transplant team.

from south africa is dr. pollack, exhibiting
a distinct brogue as he speaks.
diminutive, soft-spoken, and
attired in polyester shirt and pants
with a wide-floral tie, he
reveals a brilliant grasp of the
entire transplant process. dr. pollack
creates a simplistic, but articulate, '
picture for the patient facing life-
and-death surgery and for the
family members. if someone were to
notice this nondescript man walking
down the street, he or she would at most
believe pollack to be insignificant
in the affairs and destinies of people.

finally stands dr. benedetti. with
dark, penetrating eyes, and attired

always in hospital scrubs, this
physician on the transplant team
comes from old italy. as with the
others, dr. benedetti moves with
quiet precision through the
hospital corridors. a devout roman
catholic, he appears to grasp the
majesty of God's sovereignty.

four doctors. irish catholic, italian
catholic, south african, and black.

not one of them ostentatious. not one
dressed for success. not one demanding
an audience. pooled by God from
a cross section of cultures and
continents. created by the
omnipotent Lord . . . handpicked . . .
to intervene for david in the transplant process.

these doctors were consciously aware
that God is the ultimate Inventor
and Creator.

that they were His
tools, divinely positioned. not
mediocre. not self-seeking. one of
the most renowned teams in
the world.

this is not a group of doctors
    where each one's ego is on the line . . .
    where each aspires to fame and
    greatness. this team functions
    as one with no concern for heroics.
    each doctor does what he or she can
    do best, with reverent respect for
    the others' roles. God always
    works that way.

a liver transplant costs close to
    a half million dollars. in recovery,
    high doses of antirejection medicines
    cost hundreds of dollars a
    month. david came into this
    journey with very little medical
    insurance. living with his wife,
    connie, and their two children on
    a minister's salary made all
    the medical expenses appear
    discouraging and impossible. yet,
    for the God of *all* cattle on
    all the hills of the world, it
    meant nothing. He commands the
    cattle, and He directs the courses
    of our lives.

david approached 1996 with trepidation
 and grave fear. God did for
 him what he never could have
 orchestrated for
 himself. he found a freedom
 and a new hope. in pools of
 grace, God led him through a vale
 of sorrow to the other side.

invincible. strong. God's purposes
 for his life were yet to be completely
 fulfilled.

His plans for our lives are the same . . .
 wide-open caverns of experiences and
 winding paths . . . all with potential
 to test and reveal God's Divine
 purposes for anyone, anywhere.

driving down the freeway in
 a pickup truck, david and his son,
 zachary, were quiet. david became
 so ill he had to pull off the road.
 midnight blackness. david crawled

out and began to throw up
black liquid. something he had
never done before.

he learned his liver failure had
caused the spleen to double in
size, with his blood flow backing
up into his esophagus.

it was time for david to check
himself into the hospital. october 31st.
assuming it would be only a couple
of weeks before a liver would be
available, and the transplant
behind him. great timing, he
thought. I will be back in
time for Thanksgiving and our
church's annual Thanksgiving dinner.
the first week came and went.
the second week. the third week.
if the surgery could be this week,
he could have a record recovery
and still get home by Thanksgiving.
his agitation was rising.

If we could see beyond today
        as God can see,
    If all the clouds should roll away,
        the shadows flee,
O'er present griefs we would not fret,
        each trial we would soon forget;
    For many joys are waiting yet
        for you and me.

If we could know beyond today
        as God doth know,
    Why dearest treasures pass away
        and tears must flow,
And why the darkness leads to light,
        why dreary days will soon grow bright
    Someday life's wrongs will be made right;
        faith tells us so.

If we could see, if we could know,
        we often say;
    But God in love a veil doth throw
        across our way.
We cannot see what lies before,
        and so we cling to Him the more.
    He leads us till this life is o'er.
        Trust and obey. *

*"If We Could See Beyond Today" words and music by Norman J. Clayton. ©
1943 Norman Clayton Music Pub. (A Div. of Word Music). All rights reserved.
Used by permission.

a quiet lesson that screams
through every fiber of our beings.
the lesson of patience. of giving
God time. of waiting. of realizing
that in our *best* scheme of things,
we are miles off from God's infinite,
perfect timing. our finest plans are
usually counterfeit to God's.
why is it that we rush God? that we
tell *Him* what and how things should
be rather than letting go and
finding pleasure in what we do
have at the moment?
many times, i have decided to help
God. to speed Him along. to get Him
moving in the right direction in
more expedient timing.

this is a story about God, and
God is going to do what He is going
to do. never does an infinite God
have one tiny detail off-schedule.
or a small, seemingly obscure
piece left out.

God can create circumstances to
coincide and fit together overnight,

but God is far more concerned
about the attitudes of our hearts
than He is about the magnificent
designs of our futures. His instinct
is for love. His intrinsic purity
in people's lives is to watch
events and circumstances change
everyone in a given picture.
God cares nothing about impressing
anyone with how
brilliantly, how significantly we
humans function or perform. He
only cares that a lost and
broken world be empowered by
His love and grace. and
sometimes . . . just sometimes . . .
it is more important to Him
that we be still and quiet
and wait
than that our impetuous demands
be answered overnight.
for in waiting, we are stopped
to see ourselves as we really are.
in quietness, we hear others' cries
over our own.
with prayers bouncing, seemingly
off a black sky of deafness,

God shows us secrets about ourselves
and others. secrets that warm
hearts and bring pained souls
together in comfort.
as Thanksgiving Day approached,
david realized there would be no
transplant in his time frame. the
hospital gave him an eight-hour
pass to have Thanksgiving dinner
with his family in a small hotel
close to the hospital.

*the fifth week passed in the hospital.
the sixth. david started feeling
very restless. the hospital had
become his home.*

there were tunnel systems running
everywhere through the hospital.
david started walking
through them late at night. in the
early morning hours, he would go to
rehab for workouts.

long before david ever entered the
hospital, it became clear to him

that even at 6'6" tall, he was
overweight. that it would be wise, probably,
to do his best to get into shape. for
several months, he rose before daylight
and headed for the YMCA. swimming.
weights. running. by the time he
arrived at the hospital, he was down
to what the doctors believed a near-
perfect weight.
being in the hospital now for weeks, he
was continuing his workout regimen
in any creative way he could. it
was the one thing . . . besides prayer . . .
he knew he could keep working on
in preparation for the transplant.

on one occasion, david went to see
dr. pollack, one of the surgeons. pollack's
office was in another building on
the UIC campus. as he
entered the building, he realized
the office was on the sixth floor.

impatiently, he waited for the
elevator. frustrated, he took the
stairs, not realizing the door at
the top was the one that led into

the secretary's office.
as david walked in, the secretary
looked up, startled.

"did you just climb those six flights
of stairs?" she asked in amazement.

"yes."

"you aren't even breathing hard."

"no."

"david, everyone else who comes in
is always out of breath!"

daily, he would climb the hospital
stairs from the basement to the
eighth floor . . . 109 stairs . . . 10 times
a day. he became so used to
the stairs, workouts, stationary bikes,
swimming, stair-stepper machine,
treadmill . . . until all of it became
almost an intrinsic part of the journey.

add God's spiritual preparation to
the physical readiness, and david
genuinely felt he was ready at
any given time for the transplant.

headphones on, listening to
tapes and music, david would talk
to God, and God's Spirit would
talk to him.

but now in david's seventh week . . .
hospital entombed . . . his spirits
began to spill all over the walls of
his small, tidy hospital room.
one night, specifically, lying in
bed, david began to think . . .
"God, i have to spend Christmas in
the hospital! You have taken my
family away, my church away,
i can't preach, i can't sing.
i can't even tuck my kids in
bed at night and pray with
them."

because *this is a story about God,*
i believe we must stop and all look
at ourselves.

so many times, i have despaired too.

    "God! can't You see me?

        where are You?

    God, i'm screaming. give me

    Your attention! listen to me, God!

    i cannot go on: this hurts so

    much, God . . . so, so much!"

*God is a patient Father.
a loving, compassionate,
redemptive Lord.*

He *always* hears us. *always* sees

    and cares about our frustration.

yet He is never led astray. He

    will not be hurried because the

    plans He sets in motion are

    perfect . . . the timing flawless.

and His purpose even in forcing

    us to wait . . .

    to tame our stubborn wills . . . is

    to create something gentler, more

    beautiful in our souls.

and because this is all about

    God, maybe we should

    understand right here

that wherever God is at work,
evil lurks everywhere. always.
evil can never ultimately
win for God's power is *always*
    greater. greater. greater!
but it hovers everywhere.

when God is about to perform one
    of His heart-stopping miracles, all
    the darkness of hell and evil
    attempt to thwart the power
    and destroy God's glory.
    yet His power and glory cannot be
    stopped! never!

david's despair continued.
    "God, do You know how long it
    has been since i hugged and
    kissed my wife?
    "God, You have stripped me
    of everything and all the
    loves of my life.
    i don't think this is fair!
    i don't think You understand . . .
    i am stuck in this hospital.
        waiting. waiting. hoping.
        and *nothing* is happening.

"God, if You are the Designer of life,
   can't You provide *something*
for me?

"i've put my time in for You.
   tried to adapt and make
   the best of a poor situation . . ."

no answer.
   deafening silence.
   david figured that God probably
   would just leave him in for
   another month with that
   kind of attitude.

(and God did . . . but not in anger
   or punishment. God always has a
   magnificent surprise at the
   darkest moment!)

it was during this week, december 16,
   that a man in the same condition
   as david . . . desperately needing a liver . . .
   was brought into the next hospital
   room. a professor for illinois state
      university. a ph.d.

he slipped into david's room around
    10 p.m. one night. he told of feeling a
    warm sensation. that he had noticed
    that david was a religious man.
    could david explain this to him?

david asked,
    "have you ever attended church?"

    "no," he replied.

"have you ever been associated
    with a church or Christians?"

the professor said that as a child,
    he had been to church . . . was a
    catholic . . . but had never known
    Christ or believed God was
    anything but a God of judgment.
    "ron," david continued, "you cannot go
    through something like this unless
    you have the Lord! the risks are so
    high, the odds so great. you
    need Jesus to help you through
    this. can i pray with you?"

"yes . . ."

that night, in david's room, he and
the professor prayed a simple,
childlike prayer, asking Christ to
be a part of his life. david
promised to bring his Bible the
next day and have a little
service with him.

a communion . . . a uniting . . . of
two broken, scared, troubled men
needing the God of the universe to
provide a future and a hope for
them. needing a Savior to rescue
their sinking lives.

the professor seemed delighted. he
agreed to meet. this man was
extremely critical. very jaundiced.
just to make it through the
transplant would be a long shot.
the following day, david went to
the professor's room. *Bible* in hand.
as he entered, he could see the
man was sleeping.

in fact, this man never woke up.
he lapsed into a coma, never to

open his eyes again. david was
the last one on earth to talk
to him.

thoughts came pouring in. the
professor could not walk by
himself. whenever he went to
therapy, he would always be
taken by wheelchair. he was
too weak to make it on his own.
even in bathing, he needed assistance.

david thought . . . how had the professor
walked from his bed to david's
room?

it had to be God and His angels
giving him support and strength.

*God . . . yes, God . . . brought him into
david's room.*

and david began to hear God.

"I wanted to see if you were going to
be faithful to Me . . ."

if the transplant for david had occurred

earlier, his path would never have

crossed with this man's. the professor, a

closet alcoholic with secret sins and

private failures, found God. he did

not die without hope. and he carried

with him a future in heaven.

God's incredible, all-reaching love

that is always

always

calling broken lives to His

cleansing and healing.

God's changeless power that cares

not where we have been or what

we have done. He is waiting to

set us free. there is room at the

Cross.

Tho' millions have come, there's still room for one.
Yes, there's room at the cross for you.*

david changed. he realized this

journey was not to be a self-driven,

self-absorbed, and all-consuming

mission for himself.

*"There's Room at the Cross for You" by Ira F. Stanphill. Copyright© 1946 by
Singspiration Music/ASCAP. All rights reserved. Used by permission.

his prayer life was different. he began
    to pray for others rather than
    himself. for the family who would
    be mourning because of the death
    that had to occur . . . somewhere . . . in
    order for him to receive the liver.

he prayed the donor family would be
    strengthened as he would be given
    a second chance to live.
    he prayed for the transplant team
    and the nurses.

a focus from the inward to the
    outward. from selfish to giving.
    and suddenly, everything took on a
    new perspective. when God sees
    we are listening and obedient,
    the tide begins to turn

the transplant surgeon, dr. pollack, came
    to david's room late one night. he
    explained everything concerning
    the liver transplant (the most
    difficult of all the transplant procedures).
    they visited about how long
    the surgery would take . . . the chance
    of complications . . . the amount of
    blood that would probably be transfused . . .
    and all that would be needed to
    make everything work.

david listened, quietly, for about an
    hour.

"do you have any questions, david?"

"no, dr. pollack, no questions . . . but
        i do have something to say.
    i would like you to know that i am
    a pastor of a church that is
    worldwide, and literally
    thousands are praying for this
    one surgery . . .

"dr. pollack, this surgery is going to be
    different from the rest. God will be

assisting you in a special way. the
angels will surround the operating room,
and you will sense a Presence
that you have not felt before.
you will ask yourself 'what is going on?'

*"i want you to know that God
will be there, and to not be
alarmed."*

dr. pollack thanked david and slipped
out into the night.

a brilliant surgeon, listening.
a young minister fighting
for his life . . .
and the Eternal God of the universe
preparing all the details of an
event that would not only
affect david's life for the good . . .
but reveal, clearly, the power of
Almighty God to love and
transform people as only He can.

david did not see dr. pollack again
until the day of his transplant.

Christmas came and went.

    the children and connie (david's wife)

    came to the hospital rather than

    what they all longed for . . . to be

    home around their Christmas tree.

    a real family again.

the final week of december dragged

    by. a hopeless albatross

    around david's neck.

If Jesus is the Captain of your life,
Then why can't you get through the storm?
If Jesus is the Captain of your life,
Then why do you seem so alone?
He's seen all the storms and He's ridden them through,
Though your mast and rigging are torn.
If Jesus is the Captain of your life,
Then why can't you get through the storm?*

david towered over connie,

    tiny and petite. his wife of 21 years

    was a strong person. she felt

    emotional about nature, children,

    the elderly . . . but she was not a

    weepy person. God had established

    a strong sense of self-esteem in her,

    with some definite opinions, but

    she was gentle and fun loving.

*"The Captain," words and music by Chuck Millhuff. Copyright © 1990. All rights reserved. Used by permission.

their children, zachary (14) and kaila (11),
loved to sit on her lap or snuggle
in bed with her and their dad.

six years before, when she heard
the diagnosis of david, connie
initially felt numb. she remembers
that david had turned completely
white in the doctor's office that day.

"how do people cope?" she wondered.
"how do i face the future?"

but connie's key focus through
all this was to maintain
stability for the children. to keep
everything as normal as possible.
the last thing she wanted was for
the children to get scared or
begin questioning God. after all, she
understood that though God was utterly
good, He allowed bad things to happen
in everyone's life. pain and struggle
and devastation built strength of character
and a dependence on God's grace and mercy.

then there was the church. the congregation
of people she and david ministered

to. somehow, she thought she should be
strong for them too. the weight . . . the
burden . . . wore heavy on her heart.

each week driving the two hours
into chicago to see david grew
harder and harder. keeping house . . .
being there for the church . . . the Bible
study group . . . the kids' activities . . .
teaching school . . .

"God gives me strength," she would tell people over and over.

after two months of david's
being in the hospital, it hit her
hard one day. david would not
be coming home soon!

she began to pray . . .
"Lord, i feel lost . . . empty. i need
something to hang on to. anything
to sustain me and give me
strength . . .

sitting at the kitchen table one
morning, she opened her Bible to
1 Peter 5:7-10. it was exactly

what she needed. a turning
point in her personal journey
through all this with david.

    "Give all your worries and cares
    to God, for he cares about
    what happens to you.

    Be careful! Watch out for attacks from
    the Devil, your great enemy. He prowls
    around like a roaring lion
    looking for some victim to devour.

    Take a firm stand against him,
    and be strong in your faith. . . .

    In his kindness God called you
    to his eternal glory by means of Jesus Christ.
    After you have suffered a little while,
    he will restore, support, and strengthen you,
    and he will place you on a firm foundation."

one evening, zachary had a band
    concert. after putting the children to
    bed later, she felt tormented.
    as if she would feel better if she could
    have a temper tantrum.

picking up the phone, she called her
    sister, sobbing . . . spilling out all the

pent-up emotions of frustration and
fear and despair. her sister
mentioned that a missionary in a
foreign country had just been
captured, and no one knew where
he was.

this gave connie perspective. at
        least she knew where david was.
        she knew that God would help her, and
        all people, everywhere, who were
        suffering too.

that night, connie prayed a simple
        prayer of surrender that sustained
        her.
                "Lord, when this surgery happens,
                i know it will be ok. i know
                You will see us through.
                God, You are my Father, my
                        Husband, my Counselor, my
                        Friend . . .
                You will do what You say You will do.
                Your promises are concrete and
                trustworthy."

connie's relationship with God was
        forever changed. the pain and agony

of all this had forged a quiet, rich
path through her soul.

the children had to go through their
own private sorrow and struggles
with their daddy facing a life-and-
death situation. they feared that their
daddy was going to die; that nothing
would ever be the same again.

zachary, the older of the two, became
the man of the house, feeling
responsible for his mother and
sister while his dad was away.

kaila, with her dark, flashing
eyes, had a resilience and a
simplicity about how she viewed it.

it was especially frightening for
zachary because he was diagnosed
with colitis, exactly like father's.
it was the medications taken in david's
youth that had destroyed his liver.
david had never touched alcohol.

was all this that his dad was
going through going to happen
to him, too, when he grew up?

as time passed, though, the children
were steadied by God's strength
revealed in their parents. with the
simple, childlike faith bestowed on
children by a loving God, they were
weathering the storm remarkably.
they did the only thing they could . . .
wait it out and trust God to make
it ok.

this is a story about God . . . and
God never works on individuals alone.
He always works in groups. God's love
desires all people, in all things, to be
beautifully shaped and changed by
the events of our lives. He promises
to work all things for good.
everything!
we are all like beggars, starving
for hope. for forgiveness. for mercy.
for strength. we cannot believe that God
can really love us for we have
such a hard time loving ourselves.

we feel disbelief that God's grace
    covers all our sin and doubt because
    surely we can never forgive ourselves.

       To write the love of God above
         Would drain the ocean dry;
       Nor could the scroll contain the whole,
         Tho' stretched from sky to sky.

       O love of God, how rich and pure!
       How measureless and strong!
       —Frederick M. Lehman and Meir Ben Isaac Nehorai

God's love endures every day. every moment. in our most wicked parts. through all our doubts and selfish, piteous ways.

the hospital more and more became
    david's home and world.
    his friendships grew far beyond
    the doctors and nurses on the
    transplant floor. and these
    friendships began to activate
    prayer.

on december 27, early in the morning,
    another liver patient died with

liver failure because no liver
with the correct blood type could
be found.

on december 29, another liver
transplant patient died of cardiac
arrest.

the two remaining patients were a
woman named helen and david.
the odds were not looking very
good. and in such a time as
this, God often does humorous
things.

david walked into rehab early
the next morning.

    "hi, mr. nash," one of the physical
    therapists greeted him.

"good morning . . ."

"we've been talking about you
here, mr. nash, and we know
what you do!"

david smiled.

    "what is that?"

"well, you always come to

    rehab clean, neat, friendly,

    and happy. we have decided

    you are a car salesman!"

again, david smiled.

    "i am a salesman, but it is

    not with cars. i present

      Jesus Christ."

david proceeded to tell her how

    God was working in his life.

while in rehab the next morning,

    david's name came over the intercom.

      "david nash, come immediately

    to your room."

heart palpitating, he raced toward

    the elevator. this must mean his

    time had come. a liver had been

    found.

arriving on the eighth floor,
    david looked straight at the
    nurses' station. there stood
    dr. benedetti in his surgical
    scrubs, along with dr. wiley.
    they wanted to talk privately in
    david's room.

        "we are sending you home today,
        and dr. wiley will fill in all
        the details . . ."

dr. benedetti left the room, and
    dr. wiley said she would be back
    in an hour.

david sat on the edge of his
    bed, stunned. would he *ever*
    receive a transplant? where
    was God? would they ever find
    him an organ?
    he began to pack his things and
    called connie. she assured him
    they would immediately make
    their way to the hospital, two
    hours away.

the big picture was totally
out of focus, but in david's
heart, he knew that God's plan was
always good . . . and better than
imagined up front. God does not
make any mistakes.

dr. wiley returned and began to
share with david. helen, the one
other patient waiting with david,
died during the surgery from
complications. the transplant
team felt it best to take a
three-week sabbatical. everyone
was going to take their vacations
and leave.

for two lovely weeks, david enjoyed his family and congregation. the future unknown. relinquished. surrendered.

during all this, dr. layden had
been on vacation. when he came
back home, he heard the news of the
the deaths. when he asked about

david and heard he had been
sent home, he immediately got on
the phone.

reaching david at his office that
    early Saturday morning, he asked,
        "what are you doing out of
            the hospital?"
        "well," david replied, "they released
            me because of the last two
            transplants."

dr. layden spoke clearly, and
    adamantly:
        "david, this is a high-risk
        surgery. people die, and
        we all know that. and we
        cannot save everybody.
        david, you are not
        going to die on me.
        i will be meeting with the transplant
        team this week, and we are
        gearing up again. do not get
        comfortable, for you'll be back
        here soon, and you will be
        coming in as a status one patient!"

it was that fervent, passionate
    spirit of dr. layden's that
    put him chief in command.
    that gave people like david a
    real chance at a second go-round
    in life.

shortly after, david received
    the call to return to the hospital . . .
    january 15 . . . as a status one
    patient.

dr. hodges, a physician who had
    long been a personal friend of
    david's and had first diagnosed
    his problem called:

        "the transplant team will be
        fresh and well rested, david."

this is a story about God, and
    God knows exactly what He is
    doing. in the previous months,
    david noticed that status one
    patients usually received a transplant
    within a week. david's brother, ed,
    drove in to spend a few days and
    bring encouragement.

sunday, the 21st of january, david
was allowed a pass to attend church.
he and ed enjoyed a service at
a church on the north side of
chicago. after a good meal, as they
drove back to the hospital, the
car phone rang.

9:50 p.m.
the leading transplant nurse
spoke briefly.
"david, the time has come. a
donor has been found. you need
to come back, immediately, to
the hospital. your surgery
is scheduled for 6:45 tomorrow
morning. in fact, dr. benedetti
has gone now to harvest the
organ."

*the time had come.
david had waited so long to hear
those words. so long.*

this is a story about a matchless
God. about His power to brush
miracles across darkened skies.

to care for every small sparrow.
to orchestrate our lives with
perfect precision. the Lord of
all of life, who hears every
child's prayer, and shakes
the uncertainties of our lives
to create boundaries of safety
and peace.

> . . . let the weak say. "I am strong;"
> Let the poor say, "I am rich,"
> because of what the Lord has done for us.*

yes, poor and weak and sick
and crippled . . . people from
everywhere on earth, with any color
skin, any sin or terror, and from
any walk of life
> may come to the Cross,
> may find the Good Shepherd.
anyone!

david's moment with destiny had
finally arrived. the five years.
the months. the mindless, endless
days of struggle and destitute

*Give Thanks" by Henry Smith. © 1978 Integrity's Hosanna! Music, c/o Integrity Music, Inc., P.O. Box 851622, Mobile, AL 36685. All rights reserved. Used by permission.

wanderings were culminating
on the most miraculous day of
david's life. january 22.

"Be silent, and know that I am God!"
(Ps. 46:10).
be still!
worship
celebrate.
and always remember that
God's calendar has no
mismarked dates. not even the
slightest flaw. His ways are
perfect.

david's room became a frenzy of
activity. they began to draw
several vials of blood, along with
taking his vital signs every
30 minutes. family members
were called. flights caught. a
prayer chain set in motion. as
the transplant drew near, thousands
were praying.

when david called me, my heart
stopped. still and quiet and awed.

what would it be like to be

    whisked through swinging doors

    into the cold, sterile, brightly lit

    operating room? knowing you

    might never open your eyes again?

a liver transplant! this

    was life and death, and

    many did not live to the

    other side to talk about it.

with utter reverence, i believed

    against all odds that the

    giant God i loved . . . who had

    won my heart in love forever . . .

    would bring david miraculously

    through.

Jeremiah 29:11-13:

    "For I know the plans

    I have for you,"

    says the Lord.

    "They are plans for good and

    not for disaster,

    to give you a future and a hope.

    In those days when you pray,

    I will listen.

If you look for me
in earnest, you will
find me when you seek me."

connie's mother came in to keep the
children as connie headed for the
hospital. david's brother, jim, arrived.
his sister, bev, and her husband, ken.
his parents. much emotion. tears.
prayers. everyone had waited and
prayed and longed for this
moment, but now that it had
come, there was an overwhelming
tremble in each heart.

chicago
and all surrounding suburbs
were still covered in inky darkness.
most lights out. people
were sleeping their last hour or
two before facing another day.

serafino, as always, was
already showered and shaved.

he liked rising early. getting
a head start on the world.
frankly, he enjoyed hard work . . .
his good job . . . being responsible.
he loved providing for his family.

miki rolled over and opened one
    eye. she noticed serafino rummaging
    in the closet.

"you hiding something from me?"
she chided in a tease.
"give me a kiss before you go . . ."

"miki, i am in a hurry. i got to
    head out," serafino grumbled.

"please . . ." she whimpered. "one kiss . . ."

serafino bent over and placed
    a quick, gentle kiss on miki's lips.

"see you tonight," serafino called
    as he headed for the door.

miki smiled and rolled over to
    sleep awhile longer.

one week before, while miki was
    preparing pasta for dinner, serafino had
    seemed pensive.

"i have been thinking . . . when i
    die, i want you to cremate me!"

"cremate you? Serafino, i do not
    know. what would your family say?"

"listen, miki, when i die, my spirit
    will go directly to God.
    who cares about my body?"

miki found herself feeling very
    uncomfortable with this conversation.

"serafino, why are we talking about
    this? you are not about to die!"

the conversation ended as quickly as
    it had begun.

in a liver transplant, someone
    must die for another to live. one
    life for another.

tragedy and victory, side by side.
    loss and gain.
    devastation and joy.

this is a story about God.
    how is it that this is fair?
    that God would take one life
        in order for another to have a
        chance to live?

i can only tell you how i see it.
    that in a Holy God's arrangement,
    we all have a time for joy and a
    time for tears.

in a Holy God's scheme of things,
    our days are numbered.
    but counted out carefully.
    lovingly.
    when it is time for joy, then
    bask in it. taste all the simple,
    lovely pleasures. be grateful.
    for tomorrow, joy is for another,
    and sorrow is for us.

it feels right to me that life

 must have balance. that good

 times and hard times are

 meticulously measured out, for it is

 only in the blend of both

 that we grow . . .

 that wholeness comes.

 that we know how to laugh

  with others

  and how to cry.

substance in the human heart

 is built . . . nurtured . . . so much

 more by pain and failure

 and disappointment than by

 happiness and joy. yet God, in

 infinite wisdom, understands what

 our limits are and never

 tries us more than we can handle.

 david was receiving a second

 chance to live. to walk humbly.

 to love more deeply. to comfort

 with genuine empathy. to never

 forget that one man's life was

 offered for him.

sacred life.
Holy God.
miraculous wonder.

serafino and david to become
    one in the most unusual of realities.
    david would, for the rest of his
    life, carry in his body the healthy
    liver of serafino. and every time
    he touched another with God's grace
    and love, serafino was a part of
    the ministry of kindness too.

an hour or so later,
    the phone rang.
    "miki, you need to go to the
    hospital. serafino has been
    injured on the job."

the voice on the other end of the line
    did not sound urgent. miki did
    not feel some awful dread and
    apprehension. she assumed it was something
    minor.

that cold, winter day in january 1996,
    serafino died. he had been on top a

high ladder changing a light fixture.
a coworker had been assigned to stand
at the base of the ladder and hold it
steady. for some reason, that coworker
walked away, leaving serafino
at tremendous risk. the ladder tipped,
and serafino fell to his death, landing
on his head.

this gentle, good-natured, sincere italian
died at 37 years of age. his life snuffed out
in an instant.

he had done what he always did.
miki had told him she loved him as
he went out the door, but serafino
never came home.

tragedy. an incredible tragedy.
but *this is a story about God,* and
God sees the whole picture.
He chooses when we are born and
when we die. God is a God of order.
and God never ignores a tragedy.
He is a God who decides that every
seeming devastation should be
worked for good. that in dying,
we live.

i believe God welcomed serafino and
    said, "My child, well done."
    i believe that in God's scheme of
    things, there was purpose to serafino's
    home-going. that in dying, serafino
    could do more than in living.

miki, numb and shattered both, went
    to the prayer chapel at the hospital.
    she begged God for a miracle. to save
    serafino's life.

God answered her prayer in a completely
    opposite way than what she hoped for.

God graduates us to glory where
    we can lay our burdens down.
    God is a God of perfect decisions, even
    when we can't see any purpose
    or reason about what we have
    been dealt. i believe, unequivocally,
    that more miracles are born out
    of tragedy, pain, and despair
    than all the successes and carefree
    living combined.

God handpicked serafino, for he was
    ready to go. he died in victory.

Stop all the clocks, cut off the telephone.
Prevent the dog from barking
    with a juicy bone.
Silence the pianos and with muffled
    drum
Bring out the coffin, let the mourners
    come.
Let aeroplanes circle moaning overhead,
scribbling on the sky the message
    He Is Dead.
Put crepe bows round the white
    necks of the public doves,
Let the traffic policemen wear black
    gloves.

He was my North, my South
my East and West,
My working week and my Sunday rest.

My noon, my midnight, my talk, my
    song;
I thought that love would last forever:
    I was wrong.
The stars are not wanted now; put out
    every one;
Pack up the moon and dismantle the
    sun;

Pour away the ocean and sweep up the
    wood;
For nothing now can ever come to any
    good.

              —W. H. Auden

while fiercely struggling
    to hold composure and believe for
a miracle for serafino, miki was gently
approached by laura solis from
ROBI (Regional Organ Bank of Illinois).
would she consider donating her
husband's organs so others might
find healing?

this was something she and serafino
    had never discussed. death was so
far removed from their thinking that
a decision such as this one had
never occurred to them.
miki simply requested 24 hours
to ponder it . . . to make sure that
serafino was not going to make it.
frank, serafino and miki's only
child . . . 17 years old . . . was now losing
his father early in life just as his
father had.

contemplative, handsome, straightforward
as his father, he encouraged
miki to do it.
wouldn't dad have wanted this?
even as his father, frank was
uncomplicated in his processing of
life. would this not be honorable?
a selfless gesture in a world
reeking with self-absorption and
greed.

miki also had serafino's family
to think of. all from old italy,
staunch catholics. how would
they feel?

the next day, with prayer and
a quiet peace in her heart, miki
told ROBI they could have
serafino's heart, liver, kidneys,
and eyes.

time would prove that
miki would only hear from david
and hundreds of his family and
friends. not any other recipient
of serafino's organs ever
contacted ROBI to show gratitude.

life is a mystery.
a gift many of us take for granted
day after day.
someday, each of us will die.

as david entered OR, he remembered
    it being a very large room with
    big lights and long tables covered with
    instruments.

a cold room. people very busy getting
    things ready.

dr. benedetti walked in with a black box.
    the doctor from old italy carrying
    the priceless liver of another
    italian   . serafino.

    "good morning, dr. benedetti," david greeted him.
    "good morning, mr. nash."

    "do you have it, dr. benedetti?"
    "yes, we have a good liver."

    "would you mind if we prayed?" asked david.

    "that would be fine . . ."

the entire OR came to an immediate halt
    as david prayed for the team, the technicians,
    the nurses. it was then that david
    lost consciousness, and the transplant
    began.

as simply as it had begun,
    it was over. a normal liver transplant,
    when all goes well, takes 6-8 hours.
    with complications, up to 16 hours.
    david's surgery was completed in
    4 hours.

in most transplants, the average amount
    of blood given is between 40 and 80 units.
    in david's surgery, there were no
    transfusions, which the doctors recognized
    as a miracle. a "dry run." the
    first in medical history of liver transplantation.
    when david's sick, damaged liver was
    removed to replace it with the new liver,
    no blood flowed. and when dr. benedetti
    and dr. pollack placed the last stitch,
    the blood instantly flowed and the liver
    immediately started working.

within 32 hours, david was off all
    machines, and in 48 hours, he was out

of bed, walking laps around the nurses'
station.

God had performed the miraculous
through these gifted, dedicated
surgeons. His timing was perfect.
His plan precisely accurate.

on the sixth day, david
went home, and in three weeks,
he was back in the pulpit
preaching. he was nicknamed
bishop by dr. benedetti.

God's strength.
His grace.
in our weakness, He becomes strong.
in our powerlessness, He is empowered
to take over and be glorified in
startling, thrilling ways.

our imagination of the BEST
we think God can do is lost in
the fabric of the glory He spreads
over small thoughts and human
tinkerings.

Jesus became david's song.
>when the doctors needed an instant
>guiding of the scalpel, God became
>their wisdom and hands.
>david gained some very specific
>insights that he would never forget.
>one, the hospital became his
>mission field. a place to share
>God's kindness and warmth and
>love. to remind very sick, very
>broken people that a Savior cares.

another, never take life for granted.
>every day . . . every budding flower . . . every
>gentle breeze . . . every smile is a gift.

you know, on any day death can walk into your life with its muddy boots and snatch you out of this world.

any moment, any day.
>but we all forget. we become
>lazy in our gratitude. skimpy
>in our sharing.

today, there is a family who is without
     a daddy. for in the late-night hour of
     january 21, 1996, a good man died, and his wife
     and only son made a decision to
     donate all his organs.

what was a tragic accident turned
     into a brilliant, landscaped horizon,
     something only God can do.

david learned to never take his
     family for granted. family is precious
     and ordained by God for love and
     support. he realized a community and
     friends are created by God
     to offer prayer, support,
     and camaraderie.

for david, the church is much more
     than walls and a steeple. and certainly
     not diseased by the fake and hypocritical.
     for within the walls and among the
     pews, the Spirit of God lives . . .
     and His blood covers every stain.
     His power pushes beyond the
     judgmental, who want to be the heroes,
     to the sick and sinful and
     lost . . . for Jesus came for the
     sick.

Jesus can never be taken for granted.
    for all the powers of hell cannot
    separate us from His love.

Epilogue:
    david had a burning passion
    to meet the wife of the donor. to
    thank her face-to-face. he would
    not relent or relax until,
    somehow, this took place.

however, in transplant circles it
    is clearly understood that donors
    and recipients do *not* meet.
    letters can be sent to a
    central office . . . and passed on . . .
    but no last names.
    anonymity is enforced, or
    at the most, strongly encouraged.

this was *not* acceptable to david.
    the thought of going through life . . .
        with a second chance to give and
        feel and experience and love . . .

and not being able to thank the
one who made it possible
was devastating. how
could it be harmful?

david wanted to humbly
    tell this generous and brave woman,
    now alone, that it was a very
    treasured gift that she bestowed.
    that her husband's death
    was not in vain. that in a
    unique sense, this man still
    lived on.

Mother's Day, 1997,
    this story came full circle.

david flew miki (from florida now . . .
    where serafino had always desired
    to retire) and me to
    clinton, illinois. A year
    after the transplant.
    and a celebration it was!

tears and laughter and warm sharing.
    miki spoke of good
    times and sad times

with serafino.
she and connie cried together.
locked hearts and arms . . .
one woman without her man, and
the other with hers.

one dying so the other
    could live. one who had
    once breathed and loved
    and been. the other who
    now did because of his death.

"ann, do you think miki is happy
    to be here? is the hotel ok?
    is there anything else i can do
    for her? i am struggling, feeling
    there must be something more . . .
    another way . . . to thank her better.

quietly, i tried to articulate my
    thoughts.
    "david, nothing will ever be enough
    in your heart. nothing. miki is
    without a husband and you are
    living with a future. all i think
    miki desires is for you to continue
    your gratitude for life. for you to

love and enjoy your family and
others as serafino did."

bonded for life. connie and miki . . .
    arm in arm . . . heart-to-heart.
    miki could not have serafino,
    but she felt joy that connie had
    david . . . and that kaila and zachary
    had a loving father.

again, lastly, i say . . .
    this is a story about God.
    either in life or in death.

ordinary people made extraordinary
    by God's power.

about Truth, for God is Truth,
    and facing truth sets people free.

a story about divine orchestration . . .
    people unknown to each other . . .
    zigzagging the world to cross
    others' lives and be changed

forever. God's network is a
massive web of unique
events and mind-boggling
connections.

God does the brilliant planning.
we are only asked to obey.
our yeses to Him
bring us life.
people in this story were transformed
because they said yes
to God again and again.

in the world, where there is good,
and miracles are ready to live,
evil lurks, but God *always*
wins . . .
but only if we keep saying yes.

this is a story about God's infinite love . . .
transcending . . . limitless . . . and
how it is available for you today.
no sin too great, nor failure too
humiliating. not even one's
greed or bitterness can keep
God's love from spilling through
you, and miracles will begin
to unfold.

this a story about God.

say yes.

> I'll say yes, Lord, yes
>> to Your will and to Your way.
> I'll say yes, Lord, yes;
>> I will trust You and obey.
> When Your Spirit speaks to me,
> with my whole heart I'll agree,
> And my answer will be
> yes, Lord, yes. *

*"Yes, Lord, Yes" by Lynn Keesecker. © Copyright 1983 by Manna Music, Inc., 35255 Brooten Road, Pacific City, OR 97135. All rights reserved. Used by permission

Dr. Benedetti on God at work:

With people suffering and dying all around David and while
others were getting organs, he remained steady. Everything
went so smoothly during the transplant, better than any
other time I've done the surgery. It was quite remark-
able—not a drop of blood, not a stitch out of place. It
was a beautiful perfect case. Truly a work of God.

Dr. Layden on God and being a physician:

As physicians, we are in a unique position. Decisions are sometimes very difficult. God helps me to realize that I am still
a human being. Physicians should never be judgmental
and never put themselves in a position to be God. That's
when we make bad decisions. We have to try and under-
stand how patients feel, then we begin to know who they
really are. If we deal at their level instead of being ab-
stract with them, they will see us as other human beings
instead of physicians with power. And it's only perceived
power, not real power.

Dr. Pollack on the outlook of transplant patients:

Transplant patients have been given a gift, and in that gift,
      there is no offering you can make or thanks you can give
      or materially reward. On human terms, it parallels what
      God has done for us. Through the Holy Books we learn
      these things. I look at a transplant as a form of rebirth.
      Before every surgery, I pray for God's guidance. I pray
      that He will help me do the work that is set out before
      me. The process reminds me that we must cherish each
      day we have to live, and thank God for it.

Dr. Layden on David:

David, it is obvious that you're a very religious man. It was get-
      ting close to the time when you needed a liver, and when
      you know patients as well as I do, you can sense that
      they're no longer functioning at the capacity they once
      were. At that time you begin to ask if life is worth contin-
      uing in its present quality. Patients must then decide
      whether to take the risk, knowing they may not survive.
      Even though we know that the consequences may not be
      good, the continuation of what they have now is not life.

David, you had a great ability to adjust yourself to the deterioration of your liver and continue to work and function. Over the five years that I saw you, you were at a high energy level. As the disease progressed, you adapted to each level of deterioration. Those closest to you could not see the deterioration as I could. Eventually the time came when you could not function to full capacity as husband, father, and pastor as you could the first day I saw you. What I saw in you was a strong determination and a faith in God that gave you the strength to keep on at every stage of your disease. You never gave up! I believe that God gave you that ability.

Dr. Wiley on ministry:

I sense God using me in my work. The sense of compassion I have in caring for others can only be God given. Many times we do not realize how short life is until we are staring death in the face. Sometimes God gives us a second chance and a new appreciation of the precious gift of life.

Dr. Wiley on David:

David, you had a sense of determination and faith that everything would turn out fine, and that kept us encouraged.
You also provided strength and comfort to other patients
who were quite ill and awaiting transplants.

Dr. Pollack on David:

David, during your transplant, there was no blood given. That
is very unlikely and unique. You have been given a gift.

David on being an organ donor:

Please consider organ donation as an option for yourself and
those you love. It's a gift of life.

AFTERWORD

The waiting period seemed long. The anxiety and concern that the delay would be too long, and perhaps fatal, entered my mind a number of times. A transplant experience was nothing new to me, having lived through it with my own son's double-lung transplant. I now felt some of the same concerns for my friend David.

Although he was not my son, or even a relative, I had come to love and appreciate David as though he were one of my own. He was a pastor, and I was one of the spiritual leaders of the denomination in which he served. I felt he had so much yet to offer in life that I asked the Lord to please let him continue his ministerial career. Added to this concern was his family, who would continue to need their husband and father.

What joy I knew when word was received that David's surgery had taken place and had been a success. For the second time, I found myself jubilant over the accomplishments of modern science when accompanied with prayer and faith. Throughout the entire period, David has more often than not been the one who has inspired and encouraged many of us with his positive and optimistic faith.

Now that his story is being printed, it is my hope that thousands will receive this same boost to their trust in God as have I. David's cousin, the well-known and highly respected Ann Kiemel, has put her own unique touch to the account of this healing. The result is an exciting and readable book, which I predict will receive wide acceptance.

May God's blessings accompany these pages so that readers everywhere will be encouraged to believe for the needed miracles in their own lives.

—Jerald D. Johnson
General Superintendent Emeritus
Church of the Nazarene

MIKI'S FAREWELL

Serafino,

The only time I ever saw you in

a hospital,

You lay waiting for the last

breath of life to leave.

And all the memories,

All those dreams,

All of our plans,

All of my life

left in that last breath.

I remember a very cold January 25,

Ten years to the day of my mother's

death,

When I said

Good-bye, Sonny, I love you.

Thank you for the memories.

Miki